Eight *Little* Lessons *of* Hope & Healing

by Laurie J. Beck

design 360

First published in the
United States of America in 2011 by
Design360, llc.
2117 Olde Towne Avenue
Miramar Beach, Florida 32550
www.design-360.com

ISBN: 9780984548125
LCCN: 2011932053

2011 / 5 4 3 2 1

Printed in the U.S.A.
Designed by Keri Atchley

For my mother, Loretta LaRoche,
for all the years, and all the tears...
and because you said so.

Table of Contents

Sometimes you have to invent your own miracle.

"I firmly believe you can't just cut the cancer out of you, do some chemo or radiation, and think you're done. You have to cut the cancer out of your mind. You have to live, eat and breathe positive intention. You have to find a way to forgive so that the healing can begin. You need to search every day to find serenity. And you need to make sure that you are throwing every healing modality, Western, Eastern and otherwise, that you can, at that disease in your body."

Laurie was diagnosed with not one, but two types of cancer: Non-Hodgkin's lymphoma and marginal cell leukemia. Her prognosis was grim. She was told there was no cure available and she should begin palliative care and heavy doses of chemotherapy.

After consulting with two cancer specialists, Laurie's inner voice directed her to seek the advice of one more doctor. He suggested "watchful waiting," to wait on the chemotherapy against the advice of the previous doctors. Faced with the dilemma of differing opinions, Laurie had to make the decision of a lifetime.

She chose to wait and face the enemy cancer with love, not fear. Her fear gradually melted into resolve as she opened her heart to the possibilities that were life changing and life giving.

In her soon-to-be-released autobiography, *Living to Tell*, Laurie shares her personal story of healing and her life journey filled with hope, love and humor, not to mention a few unexpected emotional detours.

Today, Laurie is "cancer free." The enemy is described as "indolent" by her physicians but could recur anytime or never. This possibility has strengthened her resolve to stay well mentally, emotionally, physically and spiritually. She does this with her daily reminders of eight little lessons of hope and healing.

After completing her memoir, Laurie realized she wanted to share the life lessons that carried her through her Journey as a small, meditative book.

"I want to extend this knowledge to others and to encourage each individual to go within and find their personal healing power. I look back five years later with such gratitude that my mind and heart opened to a space and place I may never have found. Self-healing is an empowering choice and an action to bring awareness into our lives."

In this small book of intentions, Beck guides and shares some simple thoughts of intentions that may help you shift your thinking, if for only a second, minute or hour. Perhaps even for a lifetime. Physicist Albert Einstein theorized that, "Energy is thought." Subtle energy is the non-material fabric of the universe, limitless, infinite, everywhere in everything. Simply put, *you have the power!*

Tap into your inner Spirit.

"So as you open each chapter choose the message that best resonates with you at the time. I have eight powerful intentions that I have taken from my memoir. I chose these words and designed the chapters and pieces of crystal jewelry around these intentions."

Intention: being mentally focused.

Use your mental focus on the directed energy of LOVE by direct intention to create your outcome. Allow the result you are putting forth to be only positive intention.

The pieces of jewelry designed in the book go with each intention. What we are learning or seeing is that when we carry that thought or object with us, one can shift to that place. Crystals have a long list of metaphysical properties. I am going to share the general purpose of what the stone is used for and what makes that stone unique and special.

Allow your mind, heart and soul to open so that you can shift to a more harmonious place, and by doing so, relight the candle of hope and well-being.

Stone Glossary

Amazonite: A very soothing stone. It helps create a calming effect and can help correct mood swings. It helps promote confidence and joy for life. If placed on the third chakra, it can lift depression and reduce anxiety.

Amethyst: Known for its healing properties by improving concentration as well as alleviating migraines. It has a soothing, relaxing effect and helps promote healthy sleep. It is also used to treat swelling, insect bites, and acne. Buddhist monks used amethyst to help them meditate.

Blue Sapphire: It is the most effective healing stone for the nervous system. Psychologically, it strengthens the wearer's willpower and gives strength to get better. It is considered the most powerful and protective stone.

Carnelian: Helps with digestion. It encourages the formation of new blood cells. Helps with bleeding gums and helps firm the skin by stimulation through circulation. It increases zest for life while enhancing courage.

Citrine: Helps combat stress and depression and stimulates the metabolic processes of your liver, stomach and pancreas. It helps strengthen the immune system. It has a detoxifying effect on the metabolism. It symbolizes confidence.

Crystal Quartz: Natural quartz crystal is used as a cleansing stone to eliminate negative energies from other stones. It is said to amplify the powers of the stones that are used with it. It is believed to be a powerful tool for memory improvement and bringing clarity to one's consciousness. It is often used to fortify the nerves, stimulate glandular activity, reduce fevers, alleviate pain, swelling and nausea as well as aid in sobriety.

Labradorite: Psychologically, Labradorite has a calming and harmonizing effect. It also helps with disorders of the spinal column, wear and tear on the joints, and arthritis. It stimulates the imagination and improves clarity.

Lapis Lazuli:
Quiets the mind. Shelters the wearer like a shield. A good stone for blood purification and for boosting the immune system. A powerful thought amplifier and is helpful in aligning all elements of the body and mind.

Leopard Skin Jasper:
Helps stimulate and detoxify the liver, gallbladder and bladder. It relaxes tension and helps with nausea. Brings about harmony between the wearer and one's environment. It calms the wearer.

Peridot:
Strengthens breath of life and confidence. Helps one understand relationships and other realities. Alleviates depression, anger, fear, jealousy and anxiety. It releases toxins and brings them to the surface. Helps with mental cleansing and stimulates tissue regeneration.

Picture Jasper:
Has been known as the stone of "Global Awareness." It promotes brotherhood to work together to save the planet. It can be used to stimulate the proper functioning of the immune system, and can be helpful in the treatment of disorders associated with skin and kidneys.

Red Ruby Quartz: Stimulates
circulation and thus increases sexuality and fertility. Psychologically it opens the mind to beautiful things, enhances friendships and helps with lovesickness.

Rhodonite: It strengthens the possessor's
immune system and helps with allergies. It helps with phobias. It helps one keep a clear mind in tense situations. It can help with anxiety and has a stimulating effect on sexuality. Calms and feeds the soul.

Rhyolite: Assists in fulfilling your goals and
dreams, and helps you to know the right path from a soulful level. Rhyolite facilitates deep meditation and strengthens soul, body and mind. Rhyolite fortifies the body's natural resistance, gives strength and improves muscle tone.

Rose Quartz: Rose Quartz has a gentle
vibration of love for the owner. It gives inner peace and helps in all matters pertaining to love in all of its forms. It helps the user feel a strong sense of self-worth, therefore being worth love.

Smoky Quartz: Helpful in overcoming depression, nightmares and stress. Alleviates fear and anxiety; creates deep feelings, deep relaxation and lovingness. Ancients used it also to stimulate meridians, Kundalini and correct PMS/reproductive imbalances.

Tiger's Eye: This stone is a particularly effective healer for bronchial problems when applied to the navel chakra. Great for headaches and migraines. Helps lift depression.

Turquoise: Helps to speed up recovery after illness, alleviates pain and reduces inflammation. Psychologically it lifts depression and gives self-confidence.

To learn more about our story visit our website:

www.chibellajewelry.com

"Who looks outside, dreams.
Who looks inside, awakens."

~ *Carl Jung*

Breathe
Deep

Think
Strong

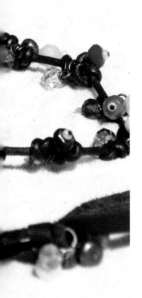

{ awaken }

{ awaken }

When we are fully awake our ability
to be present to all that is around
us increases a thousandfold!

* Learn to stop and be quiet

* Listen to your inner voice

* Become your own sanctuary

* Be in the moment

* Love yourself

* Allow yourself to feel

* Breathe five deep breaths:
  inhale/exhale from your belly

* Allow your body to relax and
  become one with your breath

In the awaken piece your grounding stone is *smoky quartz*, which is a gentle stone that instills balance, harmony and can bring peace and cleansing. *Labradorite* represents a spiritual awakening that inspires self-esteem and creativity. *Citrine* brings joy, happiness and optimism into your life. *Peridot* is an emotional healer, which also helps regulate food, diet and toxins within the body's system. *Blue sapphire* draws protection and prophetic wisdom to the user. *Amethyst* is a stone of calmness and clarity that is often used to aid in the path of sobriety.

To be fully awake is to know that you already have the answers, you know the truth. Follow that inner path and *awaken* your soul.

{ awaken }

"Where hope grows, miracles blossom."

~ *Elna Rae*

The Presence
of Today...

While Living
for Tomorrow

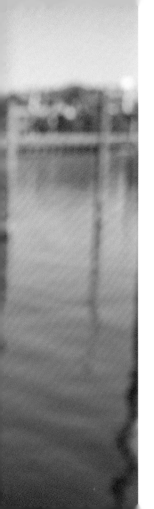

{ hope }

{ hope }

Hope endures the struggles of today and prescribes passion and motivation for a new horizon of endless opportunity.

*   Express that which you desire

*   Explore your dreams

*   Be insightful

*   Invite passion

*   Encourage hope through
    positive thoughts

Hope is expressed through the *Pearl,* which alleviates emotional imbalances and enhances personal integrity.   Pearls bring wisdom, wealth, beauty and protects one's youth. This natural stone is beneficial for the heart, lungs, kidneys and liver. Hope is the existence of today and the perseverance for a bright future.

Brown Pearl, Picture Jasper, Smoky Quartz, Citrine, Crystal Quartz

Begin each day with appreciation

and it will enhance your feelings

of *hopefulness.*

When we express our lives

with exclamations of *hope,*

we allow ourselves to know

that life is worth living!

{ hope }

"God, grant me the serenity to accept the things I cannot change, courage to change the things I can, and the wisdom to know the difference."

~ *Reinhold Niebuhr*

Peace Calms One's Presence

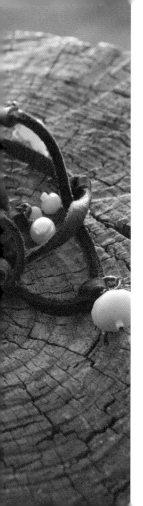

{ serenity }

{ serenity }

When your mind is free of the incessant chatter from our inner critics, we are better able to attend to being our most authentic selves and to enjoy life and all it has to offer.

* Quiet the mind

* Practice relaxed breathing

* Be still

* Embrace serene thoughts
  and release sorrow

* Stretch the body

* Invite a positive mood
  for the day

The intention of Serenity is signified through the gemstone *Amazonite,* which has a soothing affect on our nervous system and brain. Amazonite helps calm emotional and mental turmoil. This beautiful, natural stone promotes courage of personal expression and alleviates stress and exhaustion.

Amazonite, Labradorite,
Smoky Quartz
Crystal Quartz

A calm intention can attract

gathered thoughts.

Create the intention of *serenity*

and the atmosphere will follow.

The body is calmed with every breath.

{ serenity }

"Healing is a matter of time, but it is sometimes also a matter of opportunity."

~ *Hippocrates*

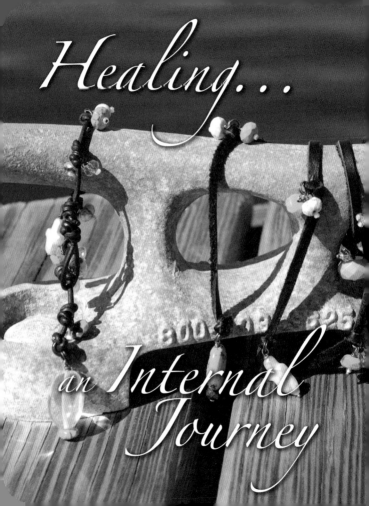

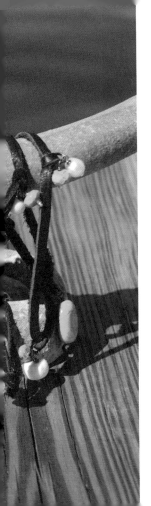

{ healing }

{ healing }

Fear is the greatest deterrent to healing, so surround yourself with a white light and begin!

* Think whole rather
  than in portions

* Overcome fear

* Embrace the gift
  of healing energies

* Be patient... Be enduring...

* Allow and embrace
  the support of others

* Forgive

* Repair the story...
  Our cells listen to ourselves

Healing is portrayed through *Turquoise*, which has powerful healing properties that benefit the mind and body. *Turquoise* has healing properties that strengthens the immune system, respiratory, waste and skeletal systems within the body. With healing comes a period of 'watchful waiting' and the prescribed *Turquoise* can protect against negative energies and bring peace to one's home.

Turquoise, Crystal Quartz, Pearl

Healing begins in the heart

and resonates through the body.

Healing oneself takes courage

and inspires others to take hold

of that which encourages strength

and humility.

{ healing }

"If you change the way you look at things, the things you look at change."

~ *Dr. Wayne Dyer*

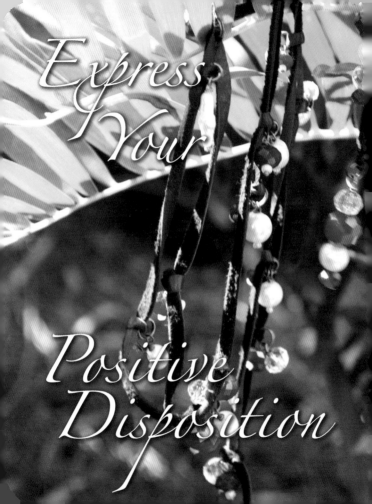

Express Your
Your
Positive
Disposition

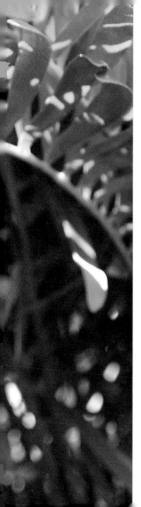

{ positivity }

{ positivity }

Even the smallest positive thought
can lead to greatness!

* Be open in your thoughts

* Show strength in adversity

* Ponder on that
  which brings joy

* See the glass half full in
  every situation

* Shift your "stinking thinking"

Positivity is expressed through the vibrant *Red Ruby Quartz*, which is a powerful stone of optimism and passion. *Red Ruby Quartz* has a stabilizing effect between passion and anger. This stone of passion and creativity allows the infusion of positive energies to flow through the body and resonate outwardly!

Red Ruby Quartz, Pearl, Crystal Quartz

Discover the benefits and

blessings of seeing the world

as if it is filled with possibilities.

Think abundance, not scarcity.

Positivity is the guide that takes

our hand and leads us down the path

toward a life filled with optimism, joy

and prosperity.

{ positivity }

"It's the soul's duty to be loyal to its own desires. It must abandon itself to its master passion."

~ Rebecca West

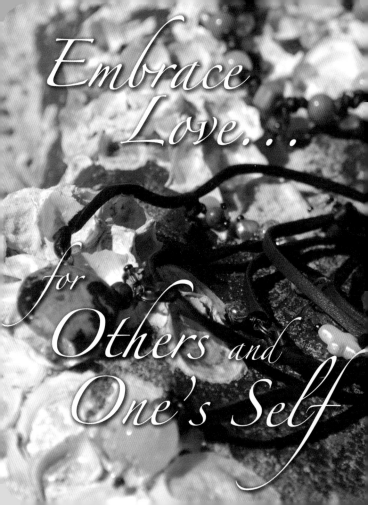

Embrace Love...

for Others and One's Self

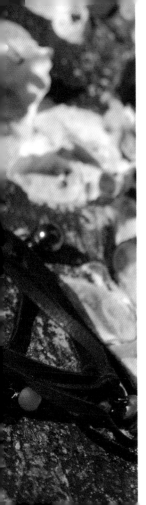

{ passion }

{ passion }

With passion in our hearts we foster
the ability to remain calm in times
of turmoil and bring resolution in a
loving way.

* Express self-affirmation

* Be optimistic in opportunity

* Prescribe love in all that you do

* Express yourself with no
  barrier to greatness

The *Rose Quartz* in the Passion piece promotes love for others and for one's self. As our physical body must heal, so must our emotions. The intention of Passion embraces self-affirmation and self-love. With passion in our hearts we foster the ability to remain calm in times of turmoil and bring resolution in loving way!

Rhodonite, Crystal Quartz
Leopard Skin Jasper,
Rose Quartz

Passion is the warm

and caring touch that promotes

peace, forgiveness and motivation.

Having *passion* in life

is the path to ensuring success.

Passion is the source

of our finest moments.

{ passion }

Awaken Your Soul

"Courage is like love;
it must have hope for nourishment."

~ Napoleon Hollingworth

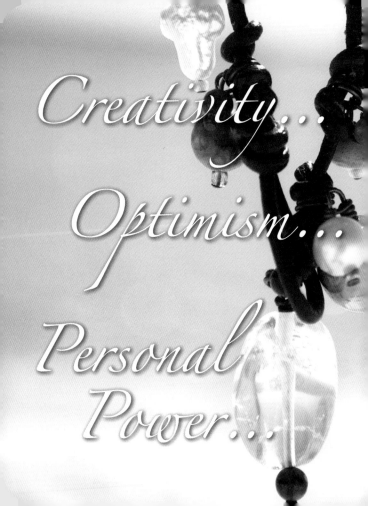

Creativity...

Optimism...

Personal
Power...

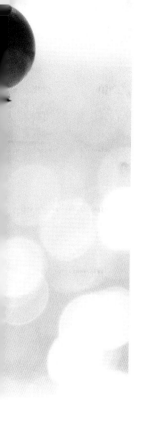

{ courage }

{ courage }

Courage is the strength that unites our energies and allows us to achieve the goals that God has intended.

* Walk outside of your comfort zone

* Confront fear

* Be scared, but press on

* Allow confidence and positive energies to guide you

* Explore your thoughts

* Have faith

Courage represented by *Rhyolite* assists in fulfilling your goals and dreams and helps you to know the right path from a soulful level. Courage is the strength to see past the trials of today and invest in hope for a brighter future. *Rhyolite* fortifies the body's natural resistance, gives strength, unites our energies and allows us to achieve the goals that inner Spirit has intended!

Rhyolite, Citrine, Labradorite, Smoky Quartz, Autumn Jasper

He who dares nothing,

need hope for nothing!

Courage impacts

the soul by surpassing

the boundaries of the mind.

{ courage }

"A sense of Humor...is needed armor. Joy in one's heart and some laughter on one's lips is a sign that the person down deep has a pretty good grasp of life."

~ *Hugh Sidney*

Originality...
Uniqueness...
Enlightenment.

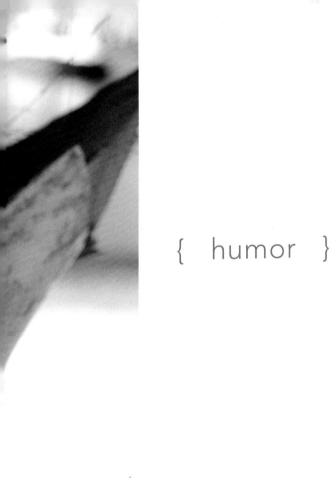

{ humor }

{ humor }

Humor stimulates the energy of love and joy by enlightening the soul to dream big and attain the impossible.

* Laugh to reward yourself

* Engage in light activities

* Take time to notice
  the smallest gifts of life

* Be the fun you're seeking

Carnelian allows energy to flow through the body, helps give a sense of humor and calms the temper. With humor in our lives we encourage the stabilizing effects that bring about greater peace and self-determination.

*Carnelian, Citrine,
Lapis Lazuli, Adventurine,
Amethyst, Labradorite,
Peridot, Crystal Quartz
Hemalyke, Tiger's Eye*

Humor allows one

to express originality

and uniqueness in a positive way.

With *humor* expressed within us,

laughter and joy resonate through our

bodies and is expressed outwardly to

impact the mood of others.

{ humor }

Acknowledgements

To the Amazing Women that made this all happen and my Knight in shining armo

Mom, this little book was truly inspired you. I have said this many times, and no it is forever written. You gave me life ar you saved my life. I am forever grateful f you and for your guidance through this am proud to be your only daughter! To n dear little darling Kaymleh, you are such gift, not just to me but to the Universe. Keri and Tricia, thank you for your amazir insight and vision and seeing what I cou not. To Gemma, for her ongoing creativi and vision of Chibella. To Lisa and Shei your talent for photography is beyo my expectations! To Judy, thank you your friendship with "edit-benefits." M importantly, my Bob, for his suppo love and constant encouragement. I thankful for all of you. Love, Lolo

Awaken Your Soul